BEAT

OBESITY TODAY

RECIPE BOOK

ACHIEVE WEIGHT LOSS AND SUPERCHARGE ENERGY THROUGH THE POWER OF INTERMITTENT FASTING!

MOH LIMS

Copyright©2023 Moh Lims

TABLE OF CONTENT

INTRODUCTION

A path toward greater health is more than just losing weight; it is a transforming process that goes beyond simple physical looks. "Beat Obesity Today: Achieve Weight Loss and Supercharge Energy Through the Power of Intermittent Fasting" is your all-in-one guide to changing your relationship with food and embracing the transforming power of intermittent fasting.

In a world full of fad diets and short cures, intermittent fasting stands out as a scientifically supported and long-term strategy to weight loss and general health. This book is more than simply a collection of techniques; it is a road map to comprehending the complicated interaction between nutrition, metabolism, and the body's intrinsic ability to repair itself.

As we progress through the pages of this guide, we will uncover the fundamentals of intermittent fasting, investigating its origins, the science behind its efficacy, and the numerous advantages it provides beyond weight loss.

Intermittent fasting becomes a lifestyle that goes beyond calorie restriction, with benefits ranging from greater energy and mental clarity to enhanced metabolic health.

"Beat Obesity Today" enables you to take responsibility of your health via carefully picked recipes, evidence-based insights, and practical suggestions.

This is not a restricted diet; rather, it is an invitation to rediscover the joy of nurturing your body, giving it with the nourishment it requires while enjoying moments of purposeful fasting.

So, let us go on this revolutionary journey together, abandoning traditional dieting concepts in favor of a comprehensive strategy that nourishes not only the body but also the spirit.

Prepare to discover the secrets of intermittent fasting and observe the wonderful benefits it may provide for your health and vigor. Your path to a healthier, more vibrant self begins right now.

Vegetarian Chili

Scenario:

It's a chilly evening, and you're craving a hearty and comforting meal. You decide to whip up a delicious pot of Vegetarian Chili. Packed with wholesome ingredients, this chili not only satisfies your taste buds but also provides a nourishing and satisfying dinner for you and your loved ones.

Ingredients:

- 2 cans (15 oz each) kidney beans, drained and rinsed

- 1 can (15 oz) black beans, drained and rinsed

- 1 can (15 oz) diced tomatoes, undrained

- 1 cup corn kernels (fresh or frozen)

- 1 large bell pepper, diced (any color)

- 1 large onion, chopped

- 3 cloves garlic, minced

- 1 zucchini, diced

- 1 carrot, diced

- 1 cup vegetable broth

- 2 tablespoons tomato paste

- 2 teaspoons chili powder

- 1 teaspoon cumin

- 1 teaspoon smoked paprika

- Salt and pepper to taste

- Olive oil for sautéing

Preparation:

1. In a large pot, heat olive oil over medium heat.

2. Add chopped onion, garlic, bell pepper, zucchini, and carrot. Sauté until vegetables are softened.

3. Stir in tomato paste, chili powder, cumin, smoked paprika, salt, and pepper. Cook for 2-3 minutes to enhance flavors.

4. Add diced tomatoes, kidney beans, black beans, corn, and vegetable broth. Stir well.

5. Bring the mixture to a boil, then reduce the heat to low, cover, and let it simmer for at least 30 minutes to allow the flavors to meld.

6. Adjust seasoning if needed. Serve hot, garnished with your favorite toppings such as chopped green onions, cilantro, avocado, or a dollop of Greek yogurt.

Benefits:

1. **Nutrient-Rich:** Packed with various vegetables and beans, this chili provides a rich array of vitamins, minerals, and antioxidants.

2. **Protein Powerhouse:** Beans contribute plant-based protein, making this chili a satisfying and nutritious option for vegetarians and vegans.

3. **Heart-Healthy:** The combination of fiber from vegetables and beans, along with the absence of saturated fats, supports heart health and may help lower cholesterol.

4. **Weight Management:** High fiber content promotes a feeling of fullness, aiding in weight management and reducing overeating.

Application:

- Serve the Vegetarian Chili on its own, garnished with your favorite toppings.

- Use it as a filling for burritos or tacos for a Tex-Mex twist.

- Spoon it over baked potatoes or sweet potatoes for a comforting and filling meal.

- Enjoy it with a side of crusty bread or cornbread for a complete and satisfying dinner.

This Vegetarian Chili is not only a versatile and flavorful dish but also a perfect option for those looking to incorporate more plant-based meals into their diet.

Stuffed Portobello Mushrooms

Scenario:

Picture this – a cozy evening gathering with friends or a special dinner for two. The aroma of Stuffed Portobello Mushrooms wafts through the air, setting the stage for a delightful and savory experience.

These mushrooms, filled with a delicious combination of quinoa, spinach, and feta, make for an elegant yet easy-to-make dish that will impress your guests or elevate your weeknight dinner.

Ingredients:

- 4 large Portobello mushrooms, stems removed

- 1 cup cooked quinoa

- 1 cup fresh spinach, chopped

- 1/2 cup feta cheese, crumbled

- 2 tablespoons olive oil

- 2 cloves garlic, minced

- Salt and pepper to taste

- Balsamic glaze for drizzling (optional)

- Fresh parsley for garnish

Preparation:

1. Preheat your oven to 375°F (190°C).

2. Clean the Portobello mushrooms with a damp cloth. Remove the stems and gently scrape out the gills using a spoon.

3. In a pan, heat olive oil over medium heat. Add minced garlic and sauté until fragrant.

4. Add chopped spinach to the pan and sauté until wilted. Season with salt and pepper.

5. In a bowl, combine cooked quinoa, sautéed spinach, and crumbled feta. Mix well.

6. Place the Portobello mushrooms on a baking sheet. Brush the outside of each mushroom cap with olive oil.

7. Stuff each mushroom with the quinoa-spinach-feta mixture, pressing it down gently.

8. Bake in the preheated oven for about 20-25 minutes or until the mushrooms are tender and the stuffing is golden brown.

9. Remove from the oven and drizzle with balsamic glaze (if using). Garnish with fresh parsley.

Benefits:

1. **Rich in Nutrients:** Portobello mushrooms are an excellent source of B-vitamins and minerals like selenium, potassium, and copper.

2. **Protein Boost:** Quinoa provides a complete source of plant-based protein.

3. **Leafy Greens:** Spinach adds vitamins A and C, iron, and fiber to the dish.

4. **Healthy Fats:** Olive oil and feta contribute heart-healthy monounsaturated fats.

Application:

- Serve Stuffed Portobello Mushrooms as an appetizer at gatherings or as a side dish for a dinner party.

- Pair them with a light salad for a satisfying vegetarian main course.

- Enjoy them on a bed of mixed greens for a wholesome and nutritious lunch.

- Serve as a fancy side dish alongside grilled chicken or fish.

These Stuffed Portobello Mushrooms are not only a feast for the eyes but also a flavorful and wholesome dish that caters to various dietary preferences. They are sure to become a staple in your culinary repertoire.

Cucumber and Tuna Salad

Scenario:

On a warm summer day, you crave a light and refreshing meal that's quick to prepare. Enter the Cucumber and Tuna Salad – a delightful combination of crisp cucumbers, flaky tuna, and a zesty dressing.

Perfect for a quick lunch or a cool dinner option, this salad is a breeze to make and offers a burst of flavors that satisfy your taste buds.

Ingredients:

- 2 large cucumbers, thinly sliced
- 1 can (5 oz) tuna, drained
- 1/4 cup red onion, thinly sliced
- 1/4 cup cherry tomatoes, halved
- 1/4 cup Kalamata olives, pitted and sliced
- 2 tablespoons fresh parsley, chopped
- 2 tablespoons olive oil
- 1 tablespoon red wine vinegar
- 1 teaspoon Dijon mustard
- Salt and pepper to taste
- Feta cheese (optional, for garnish)

Preparation:

1. In a large bowl, combine sliced cucumbers, drained tuna, red onion, cherry tomatoes, olives, and fresh parsley.

2. In a small bowl, whisk together olive oil, red wine vinegar, Dijon mustard, salt, and pepper to create the dressing.

3. Pour the dressing over the cucumber and tuna mixture. Toss gently to coat the ingredients evenly.

4. Allow the salad to marinate in the refrigerator for at least 15 minutes to enhance the flavors.

5. Before serving, garnish with crumbled feta cheese if desired.

6. Serve chilled as a light and satisfying salad.

Benefits:

1. **Rich in Omega-3 Fatty Acids:** Tuna is a good source of omega-3 fatty acids, promoting heart health and reducing inflammation.

2. **Hydrating Cucumbers:** Cucumbers have high water content, aiding in hydration and providing a refreshing element to the salad.

3. **Antioxidant-Rich Tomatoes:** Cherry tomatoes add antioxidants, including lycopene, which is beneficial for skin health.

4. **Mediterranean Goodness:** Kalamata olives contribute monounsaturated fats, offering a taste of the Mediterranean diet.

Application:

- Serve the Cucumber and Tuna Salad on a bed of mixed greens for a light lunch or dinner.

- Spoon it into whole-grain wraps for a portable and nutritious meal.

- Enjoy it as a side dish alongside grilled chicken or seafood.

- Serve on toasted whole-grain bread for a delicious open-faced sandwich.

This Cucumber and Tuna Salad is not only a tasty and healthful choice but also a versatile dish that can be customized to suit various preferences.

It's the ideal solution for a quick and nutritious meal on busy days or when you're craving something light and refreshing.

Avocado and Chickpea Salad

Scenario:

Imagine a sunny day where you're in the mood for a vibrant and nutrient-packed salad that's as satisfying as it is delicious.

Enter the Avocado and Chickpea Salad – a colorful medley of creamy avocados, protein-rich chickpeas, and a zesty lime dressing. This salad is not only quick to prepare but also a refreshing way to fuel your body with wholesome goodness.

Ingredients:

- 2 ripe avocados, diced
- 1 can (15 oz) chickpeas, drained and rinsed
- 1 cup cherry tomatoes, halved
- 1/4 cup red onion, finely chopped
- 1/4 cup fresh cilantro, chopped
- 1 lime, juiced
- 2 tablespoons olive oil
- 1 clove garlic, minced
- Salt and pepper to taste
- Optional: Feta cheese for garnish

Preparation:

1. In a large bowl, combine diced avocados, chickpeas, cherry tomatoes, red onion, and cilantro.

2. In a small bowl, whisk together lime juice, olive oil, minced garlic, salt, and pepper to create the dressing.

3. Pour the dressing over the salad ingredients. Gently toss to ensure even coating.

4. Allow the salad to chill in the refrigerator for at least 15 minutes to let the flavors meld.

5. Before serving, garnish with crumbled feta cheese if desired.

6. Serve as a refreshing and nutrient-packed salad.

Benefits:

1. **Healthy Fats:** Avocados provide monounsaturated fats, promoting heart health and satiety.

2. **Plant-Based Protein:** Chickpeas are an excellent source of protein, supporting muscle health and keeping you full.

3. **Antioxidant-Rich Tomatoes:** Cherry tomatoes add antioxidants, including vitamin C and lycopene.

4. **Cilantro Detox:** Cilantro may aid in detoxification and adds a burst of freshness to the salad.

Application:

- Enjoy the Avocado and Chickpea Salad as a light and satisfying lunch or dinner option.

- Serve it as a side dish alongside grilled chicken, fish, or your favorite protein.

- Spoon it into whole-grain wraps or pita pockets for a portable and nutritious meal.

- Pair it with quinoa or brown rice for a wholesome grain bowl.

This Avocado and Chickpea Salad is not just a salad; it's a celebration of fresh and vibrant flavors that contribute to your overall well-being.

Quick, easy, and bursting with nutritional benefits, it's a go-to recipe for those looking to incorporate more wholesome ingredients into their meals.

Broccoli and Cheese Stuffed Chicken

Scenario:

Picture a cozy evening at home, and you're in the mood for a comforting yet flavorful dinner. The Broccoli and Cheese Stuffed Chicken is the perfect solution – juicy chicken breasts filled with a delightful combination of tender broccoli and gooey cheese.

This dish not only elevates a regular weeknight meal but also brings a touch of elegance to your dining experience.

Ingredients:

- 4 boneless, skinless chicken breasts
- 1 cup broccoli florets, steamed and chopped
- 1 cup shredded cheddar cheese
- 1/4 cup grated Parmesan cheese
- 2 cloves garlic, minced
- 1 teaspoon dried oregano
- Salt and pepper to taste
- Olive oil for brushing
- Toothpicks for securing

Preparation:

1. Preheat the oven to 375°F (190°C).

2. Butterfly each chicken breast by slicing horizontally, creating a pocket without cutting all the way through.

3. In a bowl, combine chopped broccoli, cheddar cheese, Parmesan cheese, minced garlic, dried oregano, salt, and pepper.

4. Stuff each chicken breast with the broccoli and cheese mixture, securing the openings with toothpicks.

5. Place the stuffed chicken breasts in a baking dish, brush with olive oil, and season with additional salt and pepper.

6. Bake in the preheated oven for 25-30 minutes or until the chicken is cooked through and the cheese is melted and bubbly.

7. Remove toothpicks before serving. Garnish with fresh herbs if desired.

Benefits:

1. **Protein-Rich Chicken:** Chicken breasts provide lean protein, essential for muscle health.

2. **Nutrient-Packed Broccoli:** Broccoli is rich in vitamins C and K, fiber, and antioxidants.

3. **Calcium from Cheese:** Cheddar and Parmesan cheeses contribute to bone health with their calcium content.

4. **Garlic Boost:** Garlic adds flavor and may have potential health benefits, including immune support.

Application:

- Serve the Broccoli and Cheese Stuffed Chicken with a side of roasted vegetables for a well-rounded meal.

- Pair it with a simple salad to lighten the dish and add freshness.

- Enjoy it alongside quinoa, rice, or mashed sweet potatoes for a wholesome dinner.

- Slice and use the leftovers in sandwiches or wraps for a tasty lunch option.

This Broccoli and Cheese Stuffed Chicken is a culinary delight that combines the classic flavors of broccoli and cheese with the juicy tenderness of chicken.

Perfect for a special occasion or when you want to treat yourself to a comforting meal, this recipe is sure to become a household favorite.

Turkey Lettuce Wraps

Scenario:

Imagine a light and flavorful meal that combines the savory goodness of seasoned ground turkey with the crisp freshness of lettuce.

Turkey Lettuce Wraps are not only a delicious alternative to traditional wraps but also a quick and satisfying option for a healthy lunch or dinner. Get ready for a burst of flavors and a delightful dining experience.

Ingredients:

- 1 lb ground turkey
- 1 tablespoon olive oil
- 1 onion, finely chopped
- 2 cloves garlic, minced
- 1 tablespoon soy sauce
- 1 tablespoon hoisin sauce
- 1 teaspoon ginger, grated
- 1 carrot, julienned
- 1 bell pepper, thinly sliced
- 1 cup water chestnuts, chopped

- Bibb or iceberg lettuce leaves, for wrapping

- Green onions, sliced (for garnish)

- Sesame seeds (for garnish, optional)

Preparation:

1. In a large skillet, heat olive oil over medium-high heat.

2. Add chopped onions and garlic to the skillet, sautéing until softened.

3. Add ground turkey to the skillet, breaking it apart with a spoon, and cook until browned.

4. Stir in soy sauce, hoisin sauce, and grated ginger. Mix well to coat the turkey evenly.

5. Add julienned carrots, sliced bell peppers, and water chestnuts to the skillet. Cook for an additional 3-5 minutes until the vegetables are slightly tender.

6. Remove the skillet from heat. Spoon the turkey mixture onto individual lettuce leaves.

7. Garnish with sliced green onions and sesame seeds if desired.

8. Serve the Turkey Lettuce Wraps immediately, allowing everyone to customize their wraps.

Benefits:

1. **Lean Protein:** Ground turkey is a lean source of protein, supporting muscle health.

2. **Vegetable Goodness:** The julienned carrots, bell peppers, and water chestnuts add vitamins, fiber, and a satisfying crunch.

3. **Flavorful Sauces:** Soy sauce and hoisin sauce provide a savory and slightly sweet flavor profile.

4. **Low-Carb Option:** Replacing tortillas with lettuce leaves makes this a low-carb and gluten-free alternative.

Application:

- Enjoy Turkey Lettuce Wraps as a light and satisfying lunch or dinner option.

- Serve them as an appetizer or finger food at gatherings or parties.

- Customize the filling with your favorite vegetables or add a spicy kick with sriracha.

- Pair with a side of brown rice or quinoa for a heartier meal.

These Turkey Lettuce Wraps are not only a healthier alternative but also a fun and interactive way to enjoy a well-balanced meal. The combination of savory turkey and crisp lettuce creates a delightful fusion of textures and flavors that will leave you satisfied and wanting more.

Cabbage and Cashew Stir-Fry

Scenario:

Imagine a quick and flavorful dinner that combines the crunchiness of cabbage with the creaminess of cashews, all infused with savory Asian-inspired flavors.

Cabbage and Cashew Stir-Fry is a delightful dish that not only satisfies your taste buds but also provides a nutritious and vibrant dining experience. Get ready for a symphony of textures and tastes in every bite!

Ingredients:

- 1 small green cabbage, thinly sliced

- 1 cup cashews, unsalted

- 2 tablespoons soy sauce

- 1 tablespoon sesame oil

- 1 tablespoon rice vinegar

- 1 tablespoon honey or maple syrup

- 2 tablespoons vegetable oil

- 3 cloves garlic, minced

- 1 tablespoon ginger, grated

- 1 red bell pepper, thinly sliced

- 1 carrot, julienned

- 2 green onions, sliced (for garnish)

- Sesame seeds (for garnish, optional)

- Cooked brown rice or quinoa (optional, for serving)

Preparation:

1. In a small bowl, whisk together soy sauce, sesame oil, rice vinegar, and honey (or maple syrup). Set aside.

2. Heat vegetable oil in a wok or large skillet over medium-high heat.

3. Add minced garlic and grated ginger to the hot oil, sautéing for 1-2 minutes until fragrant.

4. Add thinly sliced cabbage, julienned carrots, and sliced red bell pepper to the wok. Stir-fry for about 3-5 minutes until the vegetables are slightly tender but still crisp.

5. Pour the soy sauce mixture over the vegetables and toss to coat evenly.

6. Add cashews to the wok, continuing to stir-fry for an additional 2-3 minutes until the cashews are toasted and the vegetables are well-coated.

7. Remove from heat. Garnish with sliced green onions and sesame seeds if desired.

8. Serve the Cabbage and Cashew Stir-Fry as is or over cooked brown rice or quinoa for a complete meal.

Benefits:

1. **Cruciferous Goodness:** Cabbage belongs to the cruciferous vegetable family, known for its potential health benefits, including anti-inflammatory properties.

2. **Nutrient-Rich Cashews:** Cashews provide healthy fats, protein, and essential minerals like magnesium.

3. **Vegetable Variety:** The combination of cabbage, bell peppers, and carrots offers a spectrum of vitamins and antioxidants.

4. **Balanced Flavors:** The savory-sweet sauce adds depth and flavor without excessive calories.

Application:

- Enjoy the Cabbage and Cashew Stir-Fry as a quick and nutritious weeknight dinner.

- Serve it as a side dish alongside grilled chicken, tofu, or shrimp.

- Customize the stir-fry with additional vegetables like broccoli or snow peas.

- Pack leftovers into lunch containers for a flavorful and satisfying workday lunch.

This Cabbage and Cashew Stir-Fry is not only a celebration of textures and flavors but also a testament to the ease and versatility of stir-fry dishes.

Whether you're a plant-based eater or simply looking for a delicious way to incorporate more veggies into your diet, this recipe is a winner.

Shrimp and Vegetable Skewers

Scenario:

Imagine a summer evening with the sizzle of a grill and the aroma of savory marinade in the air. Shrimp and Vegetable Skewers bring together the succulence of shrimp and the vibrant colors of assorted vegetables, creating a delightful feast for family and friends.

These skewers not only promise a burst of flavors but also make for a visually appealing and healthy grilling experience.

Ingredients:

- 1 lb large shrimp, peeled and deveined
- 1 red bell pepper, cut into chunks
- 1 yellow bell pepper, cut into chunks
- 1 zucchini, sliced into rounds
- 1 red onion, cut into wedges
- Cherry tomatoes
- Wooden or metal skewers
- 3 tablespoons olive oil
- 2 cloves garlic, minced

- 1 teaspoon lemon zest

- 2 tablespoons lemon juice

- 1 teaspoon dried oregano

- Salt and pepper to taste

- Fresh parsley for garnish (optional)

Preparation:

1. If using wooden skewers, soak them in water for at least 30 minutes to prevent burning on the grill.

2. In a bowl, whisk together olive oil, minced garlic, lemon zest, lemon juice, dried oregano, salt, and pepper to create the marinade.

3. Thread shrimp, bell peppers, zucchini, red onion, and cherry tomatoes onto the skewers, alternating between ingredients.

4. Place the skewers in a shallow dish and brush them generously with the marinade. Allow them to marinate for at least 15-30 minutes.

5. Preheat the grill to medium-high heat.

6. Grill the skewers for 2-3 minutes per side or until the shrimp are opaque and the vegetables are charred and tender.

7. Remove from the grill and garnish with fresh parsley if desired.

8. Serve the Shrimp and Vegetable Skewers hot with your favorite side dishes.

Benefits:

1. **Lean Protein:** Shrimp is a low-calorie, high-protein seafood option that supports muscle health.

2. **Vibrant Vegetables:** Bell peppers, zucchini, and cherry tomatoes provide a spectrum of vitamins and antioxidants.

3. **Heart-Healthy Olive Oil:** The olive oil in the marinade contributes healthy monounsaturated fats.

4. **Low-Calorie Grilling:** Grilling adds flavor without excessive calories, making it a healthy cooking method.

Application:

- Serve Shrimp and Vegetable Skewers as a main course for a summer barbecue or outdoor gathering.

- Enjoy them over a bed of quinoa or couscous for a complete and satisfying meal.

- Pair with a refreshing tzatziki or yogurt-based dipping sauce.

- Include these skewers in a tapas-style spread for a diverse and flavorful appetizer selection.

These Shrimp and Vegetable Skewers are not just a meal; they're a celebration of fresh ingredients and the joy of outdoor cooking.

Whether you're hosting a gathering or simply enjoying a relaxing evening, these skewers are sure to elevate your dining experience with their delightful flavors and eye-catching presentation.

Sweet Potato and Black Bean Bowl

Scenario:

Picture a wholesome and vibrant bowl that celebrates the rich flavors of sweet potatoes, black beans, and an array of colorful toppings. The Sweet Potato and Black Bean Bowl is not only a feast for the senses but also a nutritious and satisfying meal that's easy to prepare.

Whether you're a plant-based enthusiast or simply seeking a nourishing option, this bowl is a delightful choice for lunch or dinner.

Ingredients:

- 2 medium sweet potatoes, peeled and diced
- 1 can (15 oz) black beans, drained and rinsed
- 1 cup corn kernels (fresh or frozen)
- 1 avocado, sliced
- 1 cup cherry tomatoes, halved
- 1/4 cup red onion, finely chopped
- Fresh cilantro, chopped (for garnish)
- Lime wedges (for serving)
- Olive oil for drizzling

- Salt and pepper to taste

For the Chipotle Lime Dressing:

- 3 tablespoons olive oil

- 1 tablespoon lime juice

- 1 teaspoon chipotle chili powder

- 1 teaspoon honey or maple syrup

- Salt to taste

Preparation:

1. Preheat the oven to 400°F (200°C).

2. Place diced sweet potatoes on a baking sheet, drizzle with olive oil, and sprinkle with salt and pepper. Toss to coat evenly.

3. Roast sweet potatoes in the preheated oven for 25-30 minutes or until they are tender and slightly caramelized.

4. In a small bowl, whisk together the ingredients for the chipotle lime dressing. Set aside.

5. Assemble the bowls by dividing roasted sweet potatoes, black beans, corn, cherry tomatoes, and sliced avocado among serving bowls.

6. Drizzle the chipotle lime dressing over the bowls.

7. Garnish with chopped red onion and fresh cilantro.

8. Serve the Sweet Potato and Black Bean Bowl with lime wedges on the side.

Benefits:

1. **Beta-Carotene Rich:** Sweet potatoes are loaded with beta-carotene, a precursor to vitamin A, supporting vision and immune health.

2. **Protein and Fiber:** Black beans provide a plant-based protein source and fiber, promoting satiety and digestive health.

3. **Heart-Healthy Fats:** Avocado contributes monounsaturated fats, which are beneficial for heart health.

4. **Antioxidant Boost:** The combination of colorful vegetables offers a range of antioxidants for overall well-being.

Application:

- Enjoy the Sweet Potato and Black Bean Bowl as a nourishing and satisfying lunch or dinner.

- Customize with your favorite toppings such as salsa, Greek yogurt, or shredded cheese.

- Prep components in advance for a quick and easy meal during busy days.

- Serve over a bed of quinoa or brown rice for added protein and fiber.

This Sweet Potato and Black Bean Bowl is not just a meal; it's a celebration of flavors and textures that come together to create a delicious and nutrient-packed dish.

Perfect for those embracing a plant-based lifestyle or anyone looking for a vibrant and wholesome option, this bowl is sure to become a favorite in your culinary repertoire.

Greek Yogurt Parfait

Scenario:

Start your day on a wholesome note or treat yourself to a delightful snack with a Greek Yogurt Parfait. This parfait layers creamy Greek yogurt with a medley of fresh fruits, crunchy granola, and a drizzle of honey.

Not only is it a feast for the taste buds, but it also provides a boost of protein, vitamins, and a satisfying crunch, making it a perfect and customizable option for a nutritious breakfast or snack.

Ingredients:

- 1 cup Greek yogurt (plain or vanilla)

- 1/2 cup granola (homemade or store-bought)

- 1/2 cup mixed berries (strawberries, blueberries, raspberries)

- 1 ripe banana, sliced

- 1 tablespoon honey

- 2 tablespoons chopped nuts (almonds, walnuts, or pistachios)

- Fresh mint leaves for garnish (optional)

Preparation:

1. In a glass or a bowl, start with a layer of Greek yogurt at the bottom.

2. Add a layer of granola on top of the yogurt, creating a crunchy base.

3. Place a generous layer of mixed berries over the granola, spreading them evenly.

4. Add a layer of sliced bananas on top of the berries.

5. Drizzle honey over the banana layer, allowing it to gently coat the fruit.

6. Sprinkle chopped nuts on the honey-drizzled bananas for added crunch.

7. Repeat the layering process if you're using a tall glass or bowl.

8. Garnish the top with a dollop of Greek yogurt, a few berries, and a sprig of fresh mint if desired.

Benefits:

1. **Protein-Rich Greek Yogurt:** Greek yogurt is a rich source of protein, aiding in muscle repair and satiety.

2. **Fiber-Packed Granola:** Granola provides dietary fiber, supporting digestive health and promoting a feeling of fullness.

3. **Vitamins from Fresh Fruits:** Mixed berries and bananas offer a range of vitamins, antioxidants, and natural sweetness.

4. **Healthy Fats:** Nuts contribute heart-healthy fats, adding a satisfying crunch to the parfait.

Application:

- Enjoy the Greek Yogurt Parfait as a nutritious and balanced breakfast to kickstart your day.

- Serve it as a light and satisfying dessert for a guilt-free treat.

- Customize the parfait with your favorite fruits, nuts, or seeds.

- Prep ingredients in advance for a quick and convenient snack option.

This Greek Yogurt Parfait is not just a delicious treat; it's a canvas for creativity, allowing you to customize layers based on your preferences.

Whether you're aiming for a nutritious breakfast, a refreshing snack, or a guilt-free dessert, this parfait is a versatile and delightful option.

Lentil Soup

Scenario:

Picture a cozy evening at home, and you're craving a warm and hearty meal that not only fills your belly but also nourishes your body.

Lentil Soup is the perfect solution – a comforting bowl of goodness made with hearty lentils, aromatic vegetables, and a blend of savory spices.

This soup is not just a meal; it's a soothing experience that brings warmth and satisfaction.

Ingredients:

- 1 cup dried green or brown lentils, rinsed and drained
- 1 onion, finely chopped
- 2 carrots, diced
- 2 celery stalks, diced
- 3 cloves garlic, minced
- 1 can (14 oz) diced tomatoes, undrained
- 6 cups vegetable broth
- 1 teaspoon ground cumin
- 1 teaspoon ground coriander

- 1/2 teaspoon smoked paprika

- 1 bay leaf

- Salt and pepper to taste

- 2 tablespoons olive oil

- Fresh lemon wedges for serving

- Fresh parsley for garnish (optional)

Preparation:

1. In a large pot, heat olive oil over medium heat. Add chopped onions, carrots, and celery. Sauté until the vegetables are softened.

2. Add minced garlic and continue to sauté for an additional minute until fragrant.

3. Stir in ground cumin, ground coriander, smoked paprika, salt, and pepper. Cook for 2-3 minutes to enhance the flavors.

4. Add rinsed lentils, diced tomatoes with their juices, vegetable broth, and a bay leaf to the pot. Stir well.

5. Bring the soup to a boil, then reduce the heat to low, cover, and let it simmer for about 25-30 minutes or until the lentils are tender.

6. Adjust seasoning if needed. Remove the bay leaf before serving.

7. Ladle the Lentil Soup into bowls. Garnish with fresh parsley if desired and serve with a squeeze of fresh lemon.

Benefits:

1. **Plant-Based Protein:** Lentils are an excellent source of plant-based protein, making this soup a nutritious option for vegetarians and vegans.

2. **Fiber-Rich:** Lentils are high in fiber, promoting digestive health and contributing to a feeling of fullness.

3. **Heart-Healthy:** The combination of vegetables, lentils, and olive oil supports heart health by providing essential nutrients and healthy fats.

4. **Immune Boost:** Garlic, onions, and tomatoes in the soup contribute antioxidants and vitamins that may support the immune system.

Application:

- Enjoy Lentil Soup as a comforting and nutritious meal on its own.

- Serve it with a slice of crusty bread for a complete and satisfying dinner.

- Pair it with a side salad for a lighter lunch option.

- Make a large batch and store leftovers for quick and convenient meals throughout the week.

This Lentil Soup is not only a nourishing meal but also a simple and versatile option that's easy to make and enjoy.

Whether you're seeking a cozy dinner or a nutritious lunch, this soup is a go-to recipe for those looking to incorporate more plant-based goodness into their diet.

Cauliflower Rice Stir-Fry

Scenario:

Imagine a quick and flavorful stir-fry that's not only delicious but also low-carb and packed with vegetables. The Cauliflower Rice Stir-Fry transforms humble cauliflower into a versatile rice substitute, creating a light and satisfying meal.

With colorful vegetables, protein-rich tofu or chicken, and a savory sauce, this stir-fry is a nutritious and delicious option for those looking to add more veggies to their plate.

Ingredients:

- 1 medium cauliflower, grated or processed into rice-like texture

- 1 cup firm tofu, cubed (or protein of choice)

- 1 cup broccoli florets

- 1 bell pepper, thinly sliced (any color)

- 1 carrot, julienned

- 1 cup snap peas, ends trimmed

- 3 green onions, sliced

- 3 cloves garlic, minced

- 2 tablespoons soy sauce

- 1 tablespoon sesame oil
- 1 tablespoon hoisin sauce
- 1 tablespoon rice vinegar
- 1 teaspoon ginger, grated
- 2 tablespoons vegetable oil
- Sesame seeds for garnish (optional)
- Fresh cilantro for garnish (optional)

Preparation:

1. Heat vegetable oil in a wok or large skillet over medium-high heat.

2. Add cubed tofu to the hot oil and stir-fry until golden brown. Remove from the wok and set aside.

3. In the same wok, add minced garlic and grated cauliflower. Stir-fry for 3-5 minutes until the cauliflower is tender but not mushy.

4. Push the cauliflower to one side of the wok and add a bit more oil if needed. Crack an egg into the wok and scramble it.

5. Add broccoli, bell pepper, carrot, and snap peas to the wok. Stir-fry for an additional 5-7 minutes until the vegetables are crisp-tender.

6. Return the cooked tofu to the wok and add sliced green onions.

7. In a small bowl, whisk together soy sauce, sesame oil, hoisin sauce, rice vinegar, and grated ginger. Pour the sauce over the stir-fry and toss everything together until well coated.

8. Remove from heat. Garnish with sesame seeds and fresh cilantro if desired.

Benefits:

1. **Low-Carb Alternative:** Cauliflower rice is a low-carb and low-calorie substitute for traditional rice.

2. **Plant-Based Protein:** Tofu provides plant-based protein, making this stir-fry suitable for vegetarians and vegans.

3. **Colorful Vegetables:** Broccoli, bell pepper, carrot, and snap peas contribute a variety of vitamins, minerals, and antioxidants.

4. **Flavorful Sauce:** The savory and slightly sweet sauce enhances the overall taste of the stir-fry without excessive calories.

Application:

- Enjoy Cauliflower Rice Stir-Fry as a light and satisfying main course for lunch or dinner.

- Serve it as a side dish alongside grilled chicken, beef, or fish.

- Customize with your favorite vegetables or protein sources.

- Make a larger batch for meal prep and enjoy it throughout the week.

This Cauliflower Rice Stir-Fry is not just a meal; it's a culinary adventure that proves healthy eating can be delicious and satisfying.

Whether you're watching your carb intake or simply looking for a creative way to enjoy more vegetables, this stir-fry is a versatile and flavorful option.

Chia Seed Pudding

Scenario:

Start your day on a wholesome note or satisfy your sweet tooth with a nutritious and delightful Chia Seed Pudding.

This simple and versatile recipe transforms tiny chia seeds into a creamy and satisfying pudding that can be customized with various toppings.

Whether enjoyed for breakfast, as a snack, or even as a healthy dessert, Chia Seed Pudding is a delicious way to incorporate omega-3-rich chia seeds into your diet.

Ingredients:

- 1/4 cup chia seeds
- 1 cup milk (dairy or plant-based)
- 1 tablespoon maple syrup or honey
- 1/2 teaspoon vanilla extract
- Fresh fruits (berries, sliced bananas, mango chunks, etc.)
- Nuts and seeds (almonds, walnuts, sunflower seeds, etc.)
- Greek yogurt or coconut yogurt (optional)
- Drizzle of honey or maple syrup (for topping)

Preparation:

1. In a bowl, whisk together chia seeds, milk, maple syrup or honey, and vanilla extract.

2. Cover the bowl and refrigerate the mixture for at least 4 hours or overnight. Stir the mixture after the first 30 minutes to prevent clumping.

3. Once the chia pudding has thickened to a pudding-like consistency, give it a good stir.

4. Spoon the chia pudding into serving glasses or bowls.

5. Top the pudding with a variety of fresh fruits, nuts, seeds, and a dollop of Greek yogurt if desired.

6. Drizzle honey or maple syrup on top for added sweetness.

7. Serve the Chia Seed Pudding chilled and enjoy!

Benefits:

1. **Omega-3 Fatty Acids:** Chia seeds are rich in omega-3 fatty acids, which are beneficial for heart health and brain function.

2. **Dietary Fiber:** Chia seeds are an excellent source of soluble fiber, promoting digestive health and helping with satiety.

3. **Protein and Calcium:** Milk and yogurt (if included) contribute protein and calcium for overall health.

4. **Antioxidant-Rich Fruits:** Toppings like berries and mango add vitamins, minerals, and antioxidants.

Application:

- Enjoy Chia Seed Pudding as a wholesome and satisfying breakfast.

- Serve it as a nutritious snack or dessert for a guilt-free indulgence.

- Customize with different toppings to suit your taste preferences.

- Prepare multiple servings for a quick and convenient grab-and-go option.

This Chia Seed Pudding is not just a treat for your taste buds; it's a nutrient-packed delight that can be enjoyed in various ways throughout the day.

Whether you're embracing a healthy lifestyle or simply seeking a delicious and versatile option, this pudding is a go-to recipe for those looking to add more nutritional goodness to their diet.

Turkey and Quinoa Stuffed Peppers

Scenario:

Imagine a colorful and nutritious meal that combines the lean protein of turkey, the wholesome goodness of quinoa, and the vibrant flavors of bell peppers.

Turkey and Quinoa Stuffed Peppers are a delightful way to enjoy a well-balanced and satisfying dinner.

With a blend of savory spices and a medley of vegetables, this dish is not only easy to prepare but also a crowd-pleaser for those seeking a wholesome and delicious option.

Ingredients:

- 4 large bell peppers, halved and seeds removed

- 1 lb ground turkey

- 1 cup quinoa, cooked according to package instructions

- 1 onion, finely chopped

- 2 cloves garlic, minced

- 1 can (15 oz) black beans, drained and rinsed

- 1 cup corn kernels (fresh or frozen)

- 1 cup diced tomatoes (fresh or canned)

- 1 teaspoon ground cumin

- 1 teaspoon chili powder

- 1/2 teaspoon smoked paprika

- Salt and pepper to taste

- 1 cup shredded cheese (cheddar, Monterey Jack, or a blend)

- Fresh cilantro or parsley for garnish

Preparation:

1. Preheat the oven to 375°F (190°C).

2. In a large skillet, cook ground turkey over medium heat until browned. Drain any excess fat.

3. Add chopped onions to the skillet and sauté until softened. Add minced garlic and cook for an additional minute.

4. Stir in black beans, corn, diced tomatoes, ground cumin, chili powder, smoked paprika, salt, and pepper. Cook for 5-7 minutes until the mixture is well combined and heated through.

5. In a large bowl, combine the turkey and vegetable mixture with cooked quinoa.

6. Arrange the halved bell peppers in a baking dish. Spoon the turkey and quinoa mixture into each pepper half.

7. Top each stuffed pepper with shredded cheese.

8. Bake in the preheated oven for 25-30 minutes or until the peppers are tender and the cheese is melted and bubbly.

9. Garnish with fresh cilantro or parsley before serving.

Benefits:

1. **Lean Protein:** Ground turkey provides a lean source of protein essential for muscle health.

2. **Whole Grains:** Quinoa is a nutrient-dense whole grain, offering protein, fiber, and essential minerals.

3. **Vegetable Variety:** Bell peppers, onions, black beans, corn, and tomatoes contribute vitamins, antioxidants, and fiber.

4. **Calcium and Protein from Cheese:** Cheese adds calcium and additional protein to the dish.

Application:

- Serve Turkey and Quinoa Stuffed Peppers as a wholesome and satisfying dinner option.

- Make a larger batch for meal prep and enjoy the leftovers for quick and convenient lunches.

- Customize the filling with your favorite vegetables or add a spicy kick with jalapeños.

- Pair with a side salad or salsa for added freshness.

These Turkey and Quinoa Stuffed Peppers are not just a meal; they're a celebration of flavors and textures that come together to create a wholesome and delicious dish.

Perfect for family dinners or entertaining guests, this recipe showcases the versatility and nutritional benefits of combining lean protein, whole grains, and a rainbow of vegetables.

Egg and Vegetable Omelette

Scenario:

Imagine a leisurely weekend morning or a quick and nutritious weekday breakfast. The Egg and Vegetable Omelette is a classic and versatile dish that combines the protein-packed goodness of eggs with a medley of colorful vegetables.

Whether you're a breakfast enthusiast or looking for a simple and satisfying meal, this omelette is a go-to recipe that's as delicious as it is nutritious.

Ingredients:

- 3 large eggs

- 1/4 cup bell peppers, diced (a mix of colors)

- 1/4 cup tomatoes, diced

- 1/4 cup mushrooms, sliced

- 1/4 cup spinach, chopped

- 1/4 cup red onion, finely chopped

- 1/4 cup shredded cheese (cheddar, feta, or your choice)

- Salt and pepper to taste

- 1 tablespoon butter or cooking oil

- Fresh herbs (chives, parsley, or cilantro) for garnish (optional)

- Salsa or hot sauce for serving (optional)

Preparation:

1. In a bowl, whisk the eggs until well beaten. Season with salt and pepper.

2. Heat butter or cooking oil in a non-stick skillet over medium-high heat until melted and hot.

3. Add diced bell peppers, tomatoes, mushrooms, spinach, and red onion to the skillet. Sauté for 2-3 minutes until the vegetables are slightly softened.

4. Pour the beaten eggs evenly over the sautéed vegetables in the skillet.

5. Allow the eggs to set for a moment, then gently lift the edges with a spatula to let the uncooked eggs flow to the bottom.

6. Once the eggs are mostly set but still slightly runny on top, sprinkle the shredded cheese over one half of the omelette.

7. Carefully fold the other half of the omelette over the cheese, creating a half-moon shape. Press down gently with the spatula.

8. Continue cooking for another 1-2 minutes until the cheese is melted, and the omelette is cooked through but still moist inside.

9. Slide the omelette onto a plate. Garnish with fresh herbs if desired and serve with salsa or hot sauce on the side.

Benefits:

1. **Protein-Packed:** Eggs provide a high-quality source of protein, essential for muscle health and satiety.

2. **Colorful Vegetables:** Bell peppers, tomatoes, mushrooms, spinach, and red onion offer a variety of vitamins, minerals, and antioxidants.

3. **Healthy Fats:** Cheese adds richness and provides healthy fats, contributing to flavor and satisfaction.

4. **Versatility:** This recipe can be easily customized with your favorite vegetables and cheese.

Application:

- Enjoy the Egg and Vegetable Omelette for a delicious and nutritious breakfast or brunch.

- Serve it with whole-grain toast or a side of fruit for a well-rounded meal.

- Customize the omelette with your favorite ingredients, such as ham, bacon, or different cheese varieties.

- Make a larger omelette and cut it into wedges for a shareable breakfast or brunch dish.

This Egg and Vegetable Omelette is not just a breakfast staple; it's a versatile and satisfying option that can be enjoyed any time of day.

With its protein-packed eggs and a colorful array of vegetables, this omelette is a delightful and nutritious addition to your culinary repertoire.

Salmon and Asparagus

Scenario:

Imagine a gourmet-style dinner that's not only exquisite but also simple to prepare. Salmon and Asparagus is a dish that brings together the rich flavors of salmon with the crispness of fresh asparagus, creating a harmonious and nutritious meal.

Whether you're hosting a dinner party or craving a restaurant-quality dish at home, this recipe is a delightful choice.

Ingredients:

- 4 salmon fillets (6 oz each), skin-on
- 1 bunch asparagus, tough ends trimmed
- 2 tablespoons olive oil
- 2 cloves garlic, minced
- 1 lemon, sliced
- Salt and pepper to taste
- Fresh dill or parsley for garnish
- Lemon wedges for serving

Preparation:

1. Preheat the oven to 400°F (200°C).

2. Place the salmon fillets on a baking sheet lined with parchment paper. Drizzle with olive oil and season with salt and pepper. Place lemon slices on top of each fillet.

3. Arrange trimmed asparagus around the salmon on the baking sheet. Drizzle with olive oil and sprinkle minced garlic over the asparagus. Season with salt and pepper.

4. Roast in the preheated oven for 12-15 minutes or until the salmon is cooked through and flakes easily with a fork. The asparagus should be tender-crisp.

5. Remove from the oven and garnish with fresh dill or parsley.

6. Serve the Salmon and Asparagus hot, with lemon wedges on the side.

Benefits:

1. **Omega-3 Fatty Acids:** Salmon is rich in omega-3 fatty acids, supporting heart and brain health.

2. **Lean Protein:** Salmon provides a high-quality source of protein essential for muscle health.

3. **Fiber and Antioxidants:** Asparagus is low in calories, high in fiber, and packed with antioxidants.

4. **Vitamins and Minerals:** Both salmon and asparagus contribute essential vitamins and minerals, including vitamin D, vitamin B12, and folate.

Application:

- Enjoy Salmon and Asparagus as a wholesome and elegant main course for dinner.

- Serve it with a side of quinoa, rice, or mashed potatoes for a complete meal.

- Customize the dish with your favorite herbs or a drizzle of balsamic glaze for added flavor.

- Impress guests by presenting the dish on a platter garnished with fresh herbs.

This Salmon and Asparagus recipe is a celebration of simplicity and sophistication. With minimal ingredients and a short preparation time, it's a perfect option for those seeking a nutritious and delicious meal without compromising on taste.

Whether you're a seafood lover or simply looking for an impressive dinner option, this recipe is sure to satisfy your palate.

Mediterranean Quinoa Bowl

Scenario:

Transport yourself to the sun-soaked landscapes of the Mediterranean with a vibrant and wholesome Mediterranean Quinoa Bowl.

This nutritious bowl captures the essence of Mediterranean cuisine, combining colorful vegetables, protein-rich chickpeas, and flavorful Mediterranean-inspired ingredients.

Whether enjoyed as a light lunch or a satisfying dinner, this bowl is a journey for your taste buds.

Ingredients:

- 1 cup quinoa, rinsed and cooked according to package instructions
- 1 can (15 oz) chickpeas, drained and rinsed
- 1 cup cherry tomatoes, halved
- 1 cucumber, diced
- 1/2 red onion, finely chopped
- 1/2 cup Kalamata olives, pitted and sliced
- 1/2 cup crumbled feta cheese
- 1/4 cup fresh parsley, chopped
- 1/4 cup extra virgin olive oil

- 2 tablespoons red wine vinegar

- 1 teaspoon dried oregano

- Salt and pepper to taste

- Lemon wedges for serving

Preparation:

1. In a large bowl, combine cooked quinoa, chickpeas, cherry tomatoes, cucumber, red onion, Kalamata olives, feta cheese, and fresh parsley.

2. In a small bowl, whisk together extra virgin olive oil, red wine vinegar, dried oregano, salt, and pepper to create the dressing.

3. Pour the dressing over the quinoa mixture and toss everything together until well coated.

4. Adjust salt and pepper to taste.

5. Divide the Mediterranean Quinoa Bowl into individual serving bowls.

6. Serve the bowls with lemon wedges on the side for an extra burst of freshness.

Benefits:

1. **Complete Protein:** Quinoa and chickpeas together provide a plant-based complete protein.

2. **Heart-Healthy Fats:** Olive oil and feta cheese contribute healthy monounsaturated fats.

3. **Antioxidant-Rich Vegetables:** Tomatoes, cucumber, red onion, and olives offer a variety of antioxidants and vitamins.

4. **Mineral-Rich:** Feta cheese adds calcium, while chickpeas provide iron and magnesium.

Application:

- Enjoy the Mediterranean Quinoa Bowl as a light and refreshing lunch or dinner.

- Make it ahead of time for a quick and convenient meal during busy days.

- Customize the bowl with additional Mediterranean ingredients such as roasted red peppers or artichoke hearts.

- Serve as a side dish for grilled chicken, fish, or lamb.

This Mediterranean Quinoa Bowl is not just a meal; it's a culinary journey that captures the flavors and colors of the Mediterranean. With a balance of protein, vegetables, and a zesty dressing, this bowl is a testament to the simplicity and deliciousness of Mediterranean cuisine.

Whether you're a fan of Mediterranean flavors or exploring a new culinary experience, this quinoa bowl is sure to become a favorite in your repertoire.

Grilled Chicken Salad

Scenario:

Picture a light and satisfying meal that combines the smoky goodness of grilled chicken with crisp, fresh vegetables.

The Grilled Chicken Salad is a versatile and nutritious dish that makes for a perfect lunch or dinner option. With a medley of colorful vegetables, tender grilled chicken, and a zesty dressing, this salad is not only delicious but also a celebration of flavors and textures.

Ingredients:

For the Grilled Chicken:

- 2 boneless, skinless chicken breasts
- 1 tablespoon olive oil
- 1 teaspoon smoked paprika
- 1 teaspoon garlic powder
- Salt and black pepper to taste

For the Salad:

- Mixed salad greens (lettuce, spinach, arugula, etc.)
- Cherry tomatoes, halved
- Cucumber, sliced

- Red bell pepper, thinly sliced

- Avocado, sliced

- Red onion, thinly sliced

- Feta cheese, crumbled (optional)

For the Dressing:

- 3 tablespoons extra virgin olive oil

- 2 tablespoons balsamic vinegar

- 1 teaspoon Dijon mustard

- 1 clove garlic, minced

- Salt and pepper to taste

Preparation:

For the Grilled Chicken:

1. Preheat the grill or grill pan over medium-high heat.

2. In a bowl, mix olive oil, smoked paprika, garlic powder, salt, and black pepper.

3. Coat the chicken breasts with the spice mixture.

4. Grill the chicken for 6-8 minutes per side or until fully cooked and has grill marks. Allow it to rest for a few minutes before slicing.

For the Salad:

1. In a large salad bowl, combine mixed greens, cherry tomatoes, cucumber, red bell pepper, avocado, and red onion.

2. Add the sliced grilled chicken on top of the salad.

3. Sprinkle crumbled feta cheese over the salad if desired.

For the Dressing:

1. In a small bowl, whisk together extra virgin olive oil, balsamic vinegar, Dijon mustard, minced garlic, salt, and pepper.

2. Drizzle the dressing over the salad and toss gently to combine.

Benefits:

1. **Lean Protein:** Grilled chicken serves as a lean source of protein for muscle health.

2. **Colorful Vegetables:** A variety of vegetables provide essential vitamins, minerals, and antioxidants.

3. **Healthy Fats:** Avocado and olive oil contribute monounsaturated fats, promoting heart health.

4. **Light and Nutrient-Dense:** The salad is low in calories but high in nutrients, making it a

great option for those aiming to maintain a healthy weight.

Application:

- Enjoy the Grilled Chicken Salad as a light and satisfying lunch or dinner.

- Customize the salad with your favorite vegetables or add nuts and seeds for extra crunch.

- Prepare the dressing in advance for a quick and convenient meal during busy days.

- Serve the salad with a side of crusty bread for a more substantial meal.

This Grilled Chicken Salad is not just a dish; it's a culinary delight that brings together the goodness of grilled chicken and a variety of fresh, vibrant vegetables.

Whether you're looking for a healthy and light option or a quick and flavorful meal, this salad is a versatile and delicious choice.

Quinoa and Vegetable Stir-Fry

Scenario:

Imagine a quick and colorful stir-fry that combines the nutty goodness of quinoa with a variety of fresh vegetables, creating a wholesome and satisfying meal.

The Quinoa and Vegetable Stir-Fry is not just a feast for the eyes; it's a celebration of flavors and textures that makes for a nutritious and versatile option.

Whether enjoyed as a light lunch or a quick dinner, this stir-fry is a delightful addition to your recipe repertoire.

Ingredients:

- 1 cup quinoa, rinsed and cooked according to package instructions

- 1 cup broccoli florets

- 1 bell pepper, thinly sliced (any color)

- 1 carrot, julienned

- 1 cup snap peas, ends trimmed

- 3 green onions, sliced

- 3 cloves garlic, minced

- 2 tablespoons soy sauce

- 1 tablespoon sesame oil

- 1 tablespoon hoisin sauce

- 1 tablespoon rice vinegar

- 1 teaspoon ginger, grated

- 2 tablespoons vegetable oil

- Sesame seeds for garnish (optional)

- Fresh cilantro for garnish (optional)

Preparation:

1. In a large skillet or wok, heat vegetable oil over medium-high heat.

2. Add minced garlic and grated ginger, sauté for 1 minute until fragrant.

3. Add broccoli, bell pepper, carrot, and snap peas to the skillet. Stir-fry for 5-7 minutes until the vegetables are crisp-tender.

4. Push the vegetables to one side of the skillet, add a bit more oil if needed, and crack an egg into the empty side. Scramble the egg and let it cook until just set.

5. Combine the cooked quinoa with the vegetables and egg in the skillet.

6. In a small bowl, whisk together soy sauce, sesame oil, hoisin sauce, and rice vinegar. Pour the sauce over the quinoa and vegetable mixture. Toss everything together until well coated.

7. Continue cooking for an additional 2-3 minutes until everything is heated through.

8. Garnish with sliced green onions, sesame seeds, and fresh cilantro if desired.

Benefits:

1. **Complete Protein:** Quinoa provides a complete protein source, essential for a balanced diet.

2. **Colorful Vegetables:** Broccoli, bell pepper, carrot, and snap peas offer a range of vitamins, minerals, and antioxidants.

3. **Healthy Fats:** Sesame oil contributes healthy fats, enhancing the overall flavor of the stir-fry.

4. **Versatility:** This recipe is easily customizable with your favorite vegetables or protein sources.

Application:

- Enjoy Quinoa and Vegetable Stir-Fry as a light and satisfying main course for lunch or dinner.

- Serve it as a side dish alongside grilled chicken, beef, or tofu.

- Customize the stir-fry with additional ingredients such as mushrooms, baby corn, or water chestnuts.

- Make a larger batch for meal prep and enjoy it throughout the week.

This Quinoa and Vegetable Stir-Fry is not just a meal; it's a quick and flavorful journey to a wholesome dining experience.

With a balance of protein-packed quinoa, vibrant vegetables, and a savory sauce, this stir-fry is a versatile and delightful option for those seeking a nutritious and delicious dish.

Green Smoothie Powerhouse

Scenario:

Imagine starting your day with a burst of energy and a nutrient-packed drink that revitalizes your body. The Green Smoothie Powerhouse is not just a refreshing beverage; it's a blend of vibrant green vegetables, fruits, and superfoods that create a delicious and healthful concoction.

Whether you're looking for a quick breakfast, post-workout refresher, or a wholesome snack, this green smoothie is a powerhouse of nutrients to fuel your day.

Ingredients:

- 1 cup kale or spinach, tightly packed
- 1/2 cucumber, peeled and sliced
- 1/2 green apple, cored and chopped
- 1/2 banana, peeled
- 1/2 avocado, peeled and pitted
- 1 tablespoon chia seeds
- 1 tablespoon flaxseeds
- 1 tablespoon hemp seeds
- 1 cup coconut water or almond milk
- 1/2 cup ice cubes

- Optional: 1 tablespoon honey or maple syrup for sweetness

Preparation:

1. Place kale or spinach, cucumber, green apple, banana, avocado, chia seeds, flaxseeds, hemp seeds, coconut water or almond milk, and ice cubes in a blender.

2. If using, add honey or maple syrup for sweetness.

3. Blend on high speed until smooth and creamy.

4. Pause and scrape down the sides if needed, then blend again to ensure a smooth consistency.

5. Taste and adjust sweetness or thickness by adding more liquid if desired.

6. Pour the Green Smoothie Powerhouse into a glass and enjoy immediately.

Benefits:

1. **Leafy Greens:** Kale or spinach provides a rich source of vitamins, minerals, and antioxidants.

2. **Hydration:** Coconut water or almond milk adds hydration and additional nutrients.

3. **Healthy Fats:** Avocado contributes monounsaturated fats for satiety and heart health.

4. **Omega-3s and Fiber:** Chia seeds, flaxseeds, and hemp seeds are rich in omega-3 fatty acids and fiber, promoting digestive health.

Application:

- Start your morning with the Green Smoothie Powerhouse for a nutritious and energizing breakfast.

- Have it as a post-workout drink to replenish your body with essential nutrients.

- Customize the smoothie by adding protein powder, Greek yogurt, or your favorite berries.

- Make a larger batch and store extra servings in the fridge for a quick and convenient grab-and-go option.

The Green Smoothie Powerhouse is not just a drink; it's a revitalizing elixir that nourishes your body with essential nutrients.

Whether you're embracing a healthier lifestyle or simply seeking a delicious and convenient way to consume more greens, this smoothie is a versatile and flavorful option to elevate your daily nutrition.

CONCLUSION

As we approach to the end of "Obesity Today: Achieve Weight Loss and Supercharge Energy Through the Power of Intermittent Fasting," it's not just a book you've read; it's a road map you've traveled, a companion on your path to improved health.

You've studied the concepts of intermittent fasting, seen its powerful influence on weight reduction, and discovered the keys to reviving your energy levels.

As we've learned, intermittent fasting is more than just a dietary approach; it's a way of life that allows you to rebalance your relationship with food and get a better awareness of your body's natural cycles.

The path to weight loss and enhanced vitality has been illuminated by the long-term radiance of deliberate fasting times and nutritious, wholesome meals, rather than by short cures.

With the information in these pages, you're not only ready to lose weight; you're also ready to embrace a new way of life—one that aligns with your body's rhythms, encouraging longevity and general well-being.

The advantages go beyond the physical; you now have access to the mental clarity, increased attention, and improved metabolic health that intermittent fasting may provide.

Remember that this trip is entirely unique to you as you proceed. You have the skills to tailor your approach, listening to your body's signs and experiencing the pleasures of mindful eating.

Intermittent fasting isn't a hard prescription; it's an opportunity to start on a tailored adventure, figuring out what works best for you and harmonizing with the lifestyle that gives you energy.

So, go forward with assurance, equipped with the knowledge obtained from "Obesity Today." May your trip be life-changing, your days be filled with vivid energy, and your newfound happiness radiate from inside.

The route to a healthier, more powerful self is not only attainable; it is currently beneath your feet. Here's to your continuing success and overall wellbeing on this great adventure.